I0102923

A True Story of

Brain Injury and NPH Recovery

For Families and Caregivers

Copyright © 2011 Judith Powell
All rights reserved.
ISBN: 0615861083
ISBN-13: 9780615861081

A True Story of
Brain Injury and NPH Recovery

For Families and Caregivers

Judith Eileen (Jones) Powell

Edited by Verna Thornton

Belmont woman listed in critical condition

A Belmont woman who was seriously injured in an automobile accident near Morristown Wednesday is listed in "critical Condition" in the intensive care unit of the Ohio Valley Medical Center.

Judith Jones, 42 was rescued by members of the Belmont Emergency Squad. The Belmont woman had stopped breathing, but was administered cardio-pulmonary resuscitation in attempts to save her life.

She was one of several persons injured in a rash of accidents caused by Wednesday's heavy winter storm.

My Little Sister, Carol

Who miraculously performed as researcher,
physical therapist, speech therapist, occupational
therapist, and psychologist to restore me!

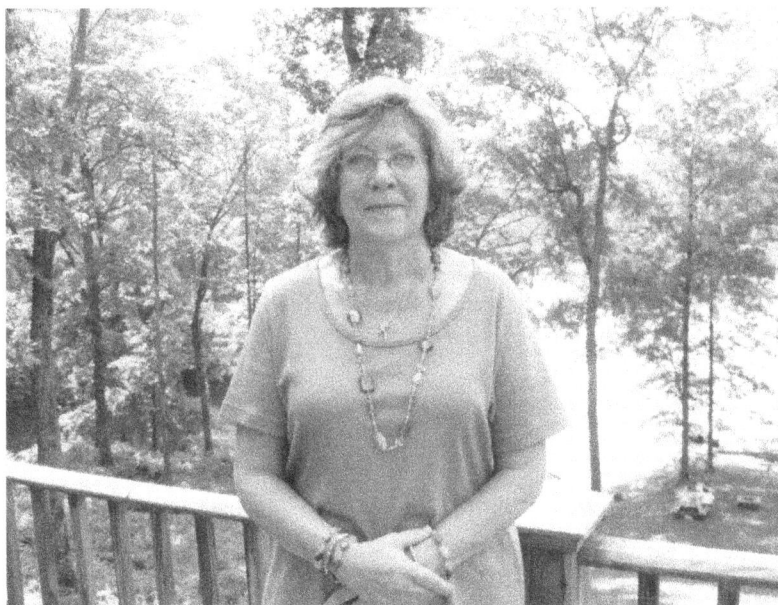

Table of Contents

Judy's Thank You

To my sister, Carol Swisk, who led me back from a "vegetable" to a fully functioning human being through her determination, creativity, persistence, and love.

To my children, Kimberly (Jones) Simon and David Jones, who taught me independence and gave me unending love and companionship.

To my parents and sister, Paul and Alice Cummins and Kathy Kell, who stood by me with total love and support.

To Julie Moore, my friend, who spent time reading to me when I was comatose.

To Wilmer G. Heceta, MD, who oversaw my hospitalization for head injury and blessed my family with his support.

To James J. Barr, MD, who referred me to a specially trained neurologist for diagnosis of NPH.

To Erick A. Arce, MD, who diagnosed NPH correctly and referred me to an appropriate neurosurgeon.

To the Shadyside High School class of 1957, which showered me with best wishes and concern.

To the writers of the Creative Writers Club of Betmar, who restored my self-confidence.

To Verna Thornton, a member of the Creative Writers Club, who voluntarily edited this book.

To Gainor Roberts, Art Curator, who transposed this book into "Word" for printing.

To the hundreds of friends and family who visited and sent cards and best wishes.

Most importantly, to my husband, Jim, who overlooked my stumbling around, fuzzy memory, and lack of coordination. He gave me his constant support, a willingness to let me "fly" alone, and his delightful sense of humor. He pushed me "just enough" and has brought me great happiness.

Endorsement

August 27, 2008

Judy Powell worked with me at the Medical Foundation of Bellaire. On January 13, 1981 I saw her dying from a car crash resulting in a severe brain injury. She lived, however, responding to our medical and her families care. She has miraculously recovered and chooses to share her success with others. I believe this book should be required reading for all rehabilitation centers and be available to all families of brain injured persons.

Wilmer G. Heceta, MD,FACS,
Diplomat, American Board of Surgery,
Diplomat, American Board of Thoracic Surgery

CHAPTER 1:

My Story

*T*his is a true story of my brain injury, its conse-
quences, and my complete recovery. I write for
the families, friends and caregivers of the 1.5 million
civilian traumatic brain injured persons each year, an
undisclosed number of war injured, and an estimat-
ed 375,000 older Americans suffering from Normal
Pressure Hydrocephalus (NPH).

I was forty-two when I suffered a severe brain injury from a head-on car collision. After three months
in a coma, it was predicted that I would permanently
remain a "vegetable" for the rest of my life. With the
help of my sister, family, and friends, I recovered and
returned to my job within one year, but it was nearly
ten years before I felt I had completely returned to
"normal."

Twenty-three years later, a consequence of my orig-
inal brain injury occurred. I developed NPH, which
caused me to become completely demented, unable
to lift my feet to walk, and unable to hold my urine.
These symptoms are often thought to be Alzheimer's

or Parkinson's disease, but fortunately, I was sent to a neurologist, specially trained in diagnosing NPH, who made the correct diagnosis and sent me to a neurosurgeon who placed a shunt in my brain. This surgical procedure brought me back to "normal," and I've been productive and happy ever since.

It is my desire to help families, friends, and caregivers of the brain-injured to understand brain injuries and learn what they can do to help their loved one recover. Insurance benefits, when available, provide only months of rehabilitation when years may be needed. These years of support have to come from family, friends, and caregivers. I hope this book provides some of the knowledge, support, and practical advice that you will need to survive your fear and lack of preparation for the task of rehabilitating your loved one.

I trust you'll enjoy the love, hope, and encouragement this book brings, describing the unexpected, humorous, positive, and sometimes miraculous happenings. Resource contact information is included.

Love and encouragement to you all.

CHAPTER 2:

A Brief Explanation of Brain Injuries

*T*he brain—what a marvelous, fascinating, complex, essential part of our being, like a thousand-piece jigsaw puzzle! Scientists have put together many pieces of the puzzle, but many pieces are still missing.

We know that separate parts of the brain control different functions. The drawing below is only a portion of what scientists know.

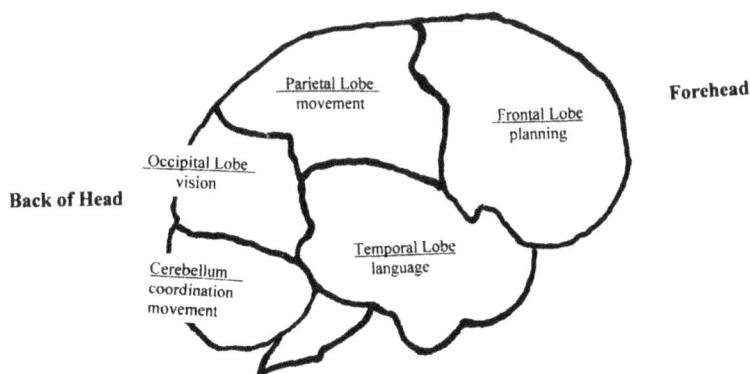

Parietal Lobe
movement

Frontal Lobe
planning

Forehead

Occipital Lobe
vision

Back of Head

Cerebellum
coordination
movement

Temporal Lobe
language

When the brain is injured, doctors can tell what parts of the brain are affected by symptoms. For example, if a person is paralyzed, the injury may be to the frontal lobe; if the person can't see, the occipital lobe may be injured. Doctors can relieve damaging pressure on parts of an injured brain, but they can't, as yet, tell us how to completely heal the brain or bring back lost functions.

Perhaps the body instinctively knows some of the answers. Most injuries and sicknesses are improved by rest. Maybe, when the brain is injured, the body instinctively puts the brain in a coma to rest. Then when the brain has rested enough, we awaken and start a new learning process like a child. Families and caregivers are like parents and informal teachers; rehabilitation professionals are like formal school teachers. It usually takes six to eight weeks to heal a broken bone, but it may take months or even years to heal a brain injury. Doctors do their best to keep us alive, and when we survive, they are elated. They have done what they were trained to do, but then the long, slow healing process begins. Insurance pays the critical portion of brain injury costs and a limited amount of rehabilitation. Families and caregivers are then left for months and perhaps years to find the finances and expertise to cure their loved ones. They need the missing pieces of the puzzle.

Because no two brain injuries are exactly alike; the rehabilitation process, recovery time, and outcomes differ with each person. Perhaps this book will provide some of the missing pieces, give comfort to families and caregivers, and provide camaraderie between us. You, the family, or caregiver can accept the role of parenting. Envision your injured loved one as a child. He or she needs your guidance, patience, instruction, encouragement, support, praise and, most of all, your love. I believe that the overwhelming love of my family gave me the impetus to live and recuperate.

Several years after surviving a brain injury, a surprise may await you. Like me, you may start forgetting things, have a hard time lifting your feet to walk, and be unable to hold your urine. You may have developed NPH (Normal Pressure Hydrocephalus), which is sometimes a consequence of brain injuries. The good news is that NPH can be effectively treated if and when it is correctly diagnosed. The bad news is that NPH might not be diagnosed correctly, and you or your family may be told that you have Alzheimer's and/or Parkinson's disease. Chapter 15 will give you the information you need to be correctly diagnosed.

CHAPTER 3:

The Accident

Count each affliction, whether light or grave, God's messen-
ger sent down to thee.
Aubrey Thomas DeVere

Another car was coming toward me. I felt my car slid-
ing and then heard a horrible, loud crunching of metal
and shattering glass.

* * *

*I*t was January 13, 1981, a cold, snowy day. I had
awakened to beautiful soft music on my clock radio
and was snuggled down under a mound of blankets,
enjoying the warmth and thinking how wonderful the
morning was. Since I divorced and my children were
in college, morning and thoughts of work were always
a pleasure.

I had become director of patient care services,
working with a wonderful group of people who, like
me, were always trying to think of ways to make our

patient visits more pleasant and our staff more satisfied. Morning was the best part of the day. The minute my feet hit the floor, I was excited, my mind whirled, and I anticipated the first pleasant "hello" of my work friends.

That morning, I stayed too long in bed, enjoying the warmth and the soft light smiling through my bedroom window, but, alas, I had to get up. The cold air hit my nightgown and, shivering, I ran for my bathrobe. It helped a little, but I couldn't wait to jump into a hot shower.

I turned the shower on to get hot while I brushed my teeth, then jumped out of my nightclothes and into the shower. Oh no! Ice! Then the water stopped. I haphazardly dried and threw my nightclothes back on, ran downstairs, and turned the sink water on. Nothing! My water pipes must be frozen.

I called my parents, who lived only a few miles from me, told them my story, and asked if I could use their shower. "Sure," my mother said. "I've got some warm blueberry muffins, so you can have some breakfast with us."

"I'll be right over."

I took my clothes with me. Bundled in my nightgown, bathrobe, underpants, heavy winter coat, and boots, I raced downstairs to my car—it groaned in the cold but kicked in, and away I went. The wheels turned slowly, lovingly crunching the snow and dimpling the smooth crust of snow covering my wide driveway. I had a hard time seeing, but knowing the landscape so well allowed me to enter the paved, two-lane road leading from my home to my father's and mother's.

Tree limbs were puffy and soft from the embellished snow. Driveways, yards, and roads were beautifully white, while snowflakes whirled in the air.

I had about three miles to go, so in anticipation of a hot shower and blueberry muffins, I traveled a little faster than I should have with unseen ice under the soft snow. Suddenly ...

* * *

As my parents waited, my mother said, "Paul, go see what has happened to her. She must be stuck in the snow." Daddy agreed and went for his car. He had trouble seeing, but he inched along slowly. A mile or so from my home, he saw a red flare, stopped his car, and walked ahead to see what had happened. His heart stopped when he recognized my car, twisted and smashed, thrust against another crumpled car. There were no police there, but a resident from a neighboring house told my father that both drivers had been taken by Emergency Squad to the hospital. Father gasped and cried out in anguish, "Please dear God, let her be alive!"

I had been rescued by paramedics and kept alive by mouth-to-mouth resuscitation as the emergency vehicle raced toward the nearest hospital. Upon arrival, I was placed on a ventilator, and holes were drilled into my skull to reduce pressure. My mother and father called Carol, my younger sister, right away. She called hospitals and found my location. They quickly went to the hospital and waited…and waited…and when they were allowed to see me, what a shock! I looked lifeless, my eyes closed, my face bruised with bandages, and tubes protruding from my head, stomach, arms, mouth, and nose. Equipment surrounding me hummed and quietly beeped. My parents could not get close enough to touch me, and my mother fell into Carol's arms, sobbing.

CHAPTER 4:

Three-Month Coma

Take rest; a field that has rested gives a bountiful crop.
Ovid

*T*he long wait began for my family and friends. I remained in a coma for three months. They didn't know if I'd live or die, and doctors gave them little hope. The rule back then for patients in an Intensive Care Unit was to allow only two people to visit for fifteen minutes each hour, so my family and friends took turns. When I became stable, although still comatose, I was moved to a step-down bed where I could be visited at any time for as long as they desired.

For their own sanity and comfort, they joined together in the waiting room. They brought candy bars, then sandwiches, cookies, and delicious homemade goodies for each other. Naturally, they shared everything with other visitors, and the waiting room became a respite of hope. The food brought smiles and moments of friendly interaction. They formed a group of comrades with the single hope that their loved ones would survive.

Family, friends, and all other visitors in ICU waiting rooms are the real "unsung" heroes—faithful to their loved ones and constantly searching for ways to help them.

It was during this time in ICU that Carol, my father and mother, my son David, my daughter Kimberly, my friend Julie Moore, and other friends initiated the help that started my healing.

Carol brought a tape player and tapes of my favorite music to play softly in my ear. She talked to family and friends about recording their voices for me, and this generated a great deal of enthusiasm. Everyone started to plan what they would say. Carol told them to say something encouraging, talk about pleasant or funny experiences they'd had with me, and express their love for me and why they wanted to be with me again. The tapes were a great success, and at Carol's request, the nurses played them or my favorite music during the forty-five minutes each hour when I was alone. The nurses were more than willing to help, and I was surrounded twenty-four hours a day with pleasant, encouraging, and loving stimulation. I believe this was the first important step in helping me regain consciousness.

For Family, Friends and Caregivers When Your Loved One Is in a Coma

It is believed that stimulation registers in the brain during inactive periods (e.g., during sleep and when a person is in a coma), so here are some steps you can take:

- Hold your loved one's hand and lovingly stroke parts of his/ her body (arms, legs, chest, back, face, and forehead).

- Play his/her favorite music. If music disturbs other patients in the room, use headphones.

- Record encouraging messages from family and friends and play them to him/her.

- Read articles, books, poetry, etc., that relates to his/her interests before the injury.

- Talk to him/her about favorite things, places, vacations, holidays, etc.

- If you sing, sing quietly.

- Express your love and assure him/her that he/ she is going to get better.

When you are unable to be at the hospital for any reason, call the hospital and ask for the nurse in charge of your loved ones' care. For military hospitals, ask for the case manager. Write down his or her name. Explain that you cannot visit your loved one, so you'd like to request the following:

- Tell the case manager or nurse that you're going to send equipment and tapes that you'd like to be played for your loved one every hour of every day.

- The tapes will include expressions of your love, words of encouragement, favorite music, voices of his/her friends, and assurances that he/ she is safe.

- The nurse will assist you in any way she or he can. Be sure to get the address and phone number where she or he can be reached to receive the items you send.

- This will not only help your loved one, it will help ease *your* mind.

CHAPTER 5:

Awakening

*Too often we underestimate the power of touch, a smile,
a kind word, a listening ear, an honest compliment, or the
smallest act of caring, All of which have
the potential to turn a life around.*
Leo Buscaglia

My eyes opened, but I seemed to be in a fog. They closed. I felt someone clasping my hand as I heard my name being repeated ("Judy…Judy"), but I didn't recognize my name. My eyes opened again and slowly began to focus. I saw color— it was pale blue— and a body. Someone was leaning over me. Where was I? Who was there? What was happening? Gradually, I distinguished a mouth and lips moving slowly. They were soft, pink and dry. While trying hard to focus on them, an unfamiliar face began to emerge, and soon I recognized Carol, my father, and my mother. My body was rigid with tension as tears began to flow. I cried, and cried, and cried. Soon, everything was dark again. A day later, my eyes opened once again to the sound of soft voices calling my name. Much to my happiness, I recognized my beautiful daughter, Kimberly, and my darling son, David. Carol and my parents were there, and I was filled with delight and joy. Tears rolled down my cheeks and drenched the pillowcase as, in my mind, I fondled the faces of my children and family. I couldn't speak, but they saw the happiness in my tears. I couldn't reach out and touch them, but they touched and kissed me.

I remained awake this time, resting only a few hours spread throughout the day, but there was a great void, like my brain had been dredged into a hollow cavity. I had no memory, no awareness of my surroundings, and no ability to reason. When not resting, I wanted to eat, and I ate all the "bad" hospital food and loved it. My family brought me scrumptious food from home and restaurants: homemade chicken and noodles, mashed potatoes, pumpkin and mincemeat pie, sweet rolls, doughnuts from the bakery, and lots of candy! After months of IV fluid and tube feedings, food never tasted so good. My thin emaciated body devoured it all like a sponge soaking up water. In the last days of consciousness in the hospital, I became happy and plump like "a right jolly old elf."

My right side was paralyzed, but physical therapists came twice a day to help me exercise in the hope that function would return. I was happier each day. I seemed to view the world for the first time in all its miraculous wonders and natural beauty. I shared that happiness with my wonderful family members, who never ceased to give me encouragement and love.

CHAPTER 6:

Going Home

*To feel the love of people whom we love is a fire
that feeds our life.*
Pablo Neruda

*H*ooray!! It was time to start my adventures—
learning to walk, read, and write, learning about
my beautiful, wonderful family—but I had no motivation. I was ecstatic just sitting comfortably in my
wheelchair, being waited on hand and foot with smiles
from everyone.

I was discharged from the hospital and sent to a
rehabilitation center where I had physical therapy,
speech therapy, and occupational therapy, but the
most enjoyable time was with my family pushing me
in my wheelchair around a courtyard in the center of
the facility. I saw and heard birds with a new appreciation, as if seeing them for the first time—how delightful! I saw a tree with its tiny leaves beginning to open,
blowing in the breeze—how miraculous it appeared
to me! I saw green grass and little purple and yellow
flowers, nodding their heads in the sunlight! It filled

me with wonder and happiness. Oh, and by the way, I still got plenty of food.

Then the work began, and I was unable to see the importance of it. I resisted physical therapy because it hurt. The occupational therapy, consisting of holding a pen and squeezing balls, was boring but tolerable. Trying to read without knowing an A from a B was so frustrating that I refused to try.

The insurance money was running out, and Carol was sad that I had shown little improvement. I could not read, write, walk, or perform the activities of daily living, but Carol had an idea that she shared with my parents and children. Everyone agreed with her idea to take me to my parents' home and continue my therapy there. After informing my doctor of their plan, I was discharged. I think that everyone at the rehabilitation center was relieved, because I had not been a very cooperative patient. In fact, I was obnoxious and still interested in only one thing: food.

I finally got to go home—to my parents' home, that is. It was wonderful being there and feeling so much love. Carol gave everyone assignments. My mother did physical therapy, exercising my legs and arms on my paralyzed side. My father supported my right side, stood me up, and encouraged me to walk. They both helped me coordinate my left side to eat, wash my face and hands, and hold a pencil. Carol came daily to check on my progress and add additional educational activities. My children were in college, but they came home every weekend and gladly helped with anything Carol suggested.

I was thrilled to be home and receive all the attention from my family. Soon, though, my childish mind figured out how to get my own way. When my mother tried to move my leg and arm, slowly but progressively each day, I figured out how to groan in pain and cry real tears until she stopped and gave me a treat. When my father tried to walk me, I made terrible faces and moaned pathetically, "Too tired." He melted immediately, sat me down, brought a blanket to cover my legs, gave me a sweet treat, and told me to relax and rest. This was blissful— I got all the sweet gooey food my stomach could hold while practicing my avoidance tactics. My life was rosy for a time.

I even duped Carol, but she finally figured out what I was doing and came up with a new plan. She decided to take me to her home and do all the therapy herself, because my dad and mom refused to be firm enough with me. Wow, did she ever meet with resistance! My mom and dad refused to consider Carol's plan. They fired, "She's our child, and we know what's best for her. We're fixing up the north wing of the house to give her a place to live out her life in peace and quiet. You know the doctors said that she'll never be able to live independently, and we're not going to inflict pain and discomfort on her. We love her and we want her to be happy. We'll take care of her. You'll not take her out of this house!"

That got Carol's dander up. She had gotten a driver's permit so she went home, got a bedroom ready for me, returned that evening with a suitcase, packed what she thought I might need, and put it in her car. She then somehow got me into her car by herself. Off we went to another "home." My parents were horrified. They threatened Carol, tried to reason with her, and my mother cried while Carol was getting me ready to leave. My father put his foot down, saying "You'll not take her!" Carol ignored them.

That night, I lay peacefully in bed, unaware of the turmoil. Carol was awake all night, praying, crying, and feeling deep remorse for the way she'd treated our parents.

The next morning, she asked our parents to come for lunch. When they arrived, she kissed them and apologized for the way she had talked to them the night before. She served a modest lunch and offered this prayer, "Dear God, please be with my dear parents and me today. May the love we have for each other bring us together in our efforts to heal Judy. You know that I believe, through You, that Judy will not live like a vegetable but rather will be whole again. Please help me, my father, and mother to do what we need to do to make this happen. Make our love for each other strong, so that we may work happily together and help each other. Thank you for your guidance, direction and love. Amen."

The family had peace and happiness again. My father and mother still had their responsibilities for my therapy, but now they were watched by Carol, who encouraged them to push me a little more each day, even when I complained and cried. Carol, bless her heart, had a sixth sense. She seemed to understand what I needed or wanted before I did. She started taking me for a ride every day to a state park near her home, which I loved. She talked to me while my mother exercised my limbs and told me what we'd see today at the park if I were able to move my leg and arm a little more than yesterday. I worked hard, because the rides had become more important than my precious food.

My father had tried to get disability for me with no success. A person at the Social Security office told him that I was able to do some form of work and therefore wouldn't be eligible for Social Security Disability. He accepted the decision and didn't pursue it further, even though it was hard for our family to make my house payments and pay other monthly debts.

For Family and Caregivers

It may take multiple requests in order to receive disability for your loved one. The following information may help you.

- Contact the Social Security Administration at 800-772-1213 or www.ssa.gov. Ask about Social Security Disability Insurance (SSDI) and Supplemental Security Income (SSI).

- If you have difficulty, contact the National Disability Rights Network Protection and Advocacy for Individuals with Disabilities at 202-408-9514 or www.napas.org.

CHAPTER 7:

Carol Forms a Care Team

*Build for your team a feeling of oneness, of dependence on
one another and strength to be derived from unity.*
Vince Lombardi

*C*arol was happy that she had me in her home,
but she wondered how she could do all that she
needed and wanted to do. How could she bathe and
dress me every day? How could she teach me to brush
my teeth and comb my hair? How could she teach me
to use a knife, fork, and spoon? Where would she find
time to teach me reading, writing, and math? What
could she do to entertain me? How could she take care
of her own children? How could she cook and clean?
Her questions raced through her mind, tumbling,
confusing, bewildering.

A plan emerged. She formed a care team by using
family and friends to divide the responsibilities. She
knew that everyone sincerely wanted to help, but for
how long? Would they know how? She called a meeting.

One weekend, these family members and friends came together at Carol's request, and they were enthusiastic and eager. Carol said, "We've all been around Judy, so we know the kind of things she needs. I'd like each of you to tell me what you see that she needs and what we can do to meet these needs." My father and mother started with the exercise programs. Some friends felt that I needed attention and companionship, so they volunteered to regularly spend time with me. My children said they'd do anything Carol thought they could do. My youngest sister, Kathy, had been unable to sit with me in the hospital because it upset her too much, but she said, "What about you, Carol? How are you going to care for your little ones? I know how I can help—I'll come every evening and weekend to spend time with them." Mother said, "And I'll cook your evening meal." On and on it went until Carol's prayers were answered, and she had her team.

* * *

Now I'd like to tell you a little about Carol, my beloved sister and healer:

Carol had no medical experience. She was thirty-two years old with a business education, married with two teenage children, and had adopted three young, mentally challenged daughters. She lived in the country with no computer or easy access to a library, and she did not drive.

The way she directed my care was miraculous. When I was comatose, she decided that I'd never be left alone and drew up a "sick-sitting" schedule. My mother and father asked to spend four hours daily with me, so Carol obliged. She scheduled my children and many friends to stay with me twenty-four hours a day. Carol was there most of every day, and she also organized the audio tapes for me.

When I came home, she had learned from physical therapists how to teach my parents to exercise my legs and arms. She took me to an indoor swimming pool daily, and I eventually overcame my paralysis. She gradually taught me to walk.

Like an occupational therapist, she taught me how to hold a fork and spoon, feed myself, use a toothbrush, and comb my hair.

Like a speech therapist, she taught me how to say letters of the alphabet, pronounce words, read words, and then sentences and stories.

Most importantly, she learned how to deal with my moods and stubbornness, my anger and temper tantrums, my game playing for sympathy and pity, and my refusal to learn. She had the wisdom of a psychologist.

* * *

Carol shared with her team what she had learned from the Brain Injury Association of America (BIAA). She wanted them to know some of the behaviors that may upset them but would pass in time. She said that I might curse, be confused, have temper tantrums, be belligerent, speak loudly, be aggressive, act childishly, or be agitated, clumsy, or irritable. She wanted them to be prepared for times when I'd refuse to do what they asked and encouraged them to be kindly persistent.

She encouraged them to give "strong" and "soft" love, saying, "You have to give Judy strong love by understanding that she has no understanding of or interest in what she needs to do to recover, so you'll often have to decide what needs to be done for her. You may have to kindly force her to do what she is capable of doing. When she doesn't want to do something, don't insist, but find ways to get her to change her mind. You can give soft love by being compassionate, patient, tolerant, and respectful. Provide assistance for her when she tries to do something but needs a little help. Encourage her to be as independent as possible. Allow her to make decisions as long as no safety risk is involved, and be prepared for advances and setbacks."

Knowing that my friends worked in the medical field, she encouraged them to talk to any professionals they knew (nurse practitioners, physical therapists, speech therapists, occupational therapists, recreational therapists, or social workers) about brain injuries. She asked them to share anything they learned with the rest of the team.

Carol gave them the information they needed in case they wanted to contact the BIAA.

For Family and Caregivers

Family and caregivers may become mentally and physically exhausted. Here are some suggestions:

- Plan relaxation times for yourselves, and make sure that they happen.

- Make time for meditation, quiet time alone, hobbies, reading, prayer, and pleasure.

- Seek out humor in movies, tapes, magazines, books. It is extremely important to have fun and laugh.

- If you believe in prayer, start a prayer chain with church members, friends, and family.

- Use the Internet to search for "Caregivers Support Groups" as well as "Help and Resources for Caregivers: Caregiving Support and Tips for Preventing Caregiver Burnout."

- Contact the National Family Caregivers Association at www.nfcacares.org.

CHAPTER 8:

Learning Adventures

*The human mind is like a piñata. When it breaks open,
there's a lot of surprises inside.*
Lily Tomlin

*I*had lost many of my faculties, but Carol ingen-
iously found creative ways to restore them. She
started with children's coloring books. The first was
an ABC Book. She taught me to recognize and say
my ABCs, one letter at a time. With an individual
letter, in large print on each page, she followed the
same routine. "Where is the letter A, Judy?" I pointed
to it with my left hand. "Say A for me, Judy." My
first attempt was "e" as in echo, but I quickly learned
to give the correct sound by imitating her. To exercise my hand, she put a bright-colored crayon in it,
and with her hand holding mine, we colored the letter
in the book. She kissed me on the cheek and praised
me for doing such a good job. At first, I didn't know
what made her so happy, but as we got to the letter F,
each time repeating all the letters up to F, I figured
out that I was doing something great. As soon as we

finished coloring the letter, I exploded with a roar of laughter and excitement. Carol proceeded to do the whole alphabet. I learned so quickly that she began to do two letters at a time, then three and more, until we reached Z. At the same time, she was teaching me small words.

It wasn't all fun and games. Often, I was completely uncooperative. When she came toward me with a book, I'd shout, "No, No, No" and refuse to do anything she asked, but boy, was she persistent. She never gave up. She never got angry and scolded me, just smiled kindly and said, "Well, I see you're not ready right now, so we'll try again a little later." I don't know what it was—her smile, her soft tone of voice, or her persistence—but I always gave in. I don't know how many hours she spent with me each day, but it had to be a lot. I started to read in about two weeks.

I had become fluent in another language—cursing—which was devastating to my family. Each day, Carol took me to a heated, indoor swimming pool to exercise my body. She put me in water up to my neck to cover my shoulders. Then she stood on one side of the pool and told me to come toward her. The buoyancy of the water allowed me to take steps and move my arm on my paralyzed side, but it was difficult. My new language served me well. I let out a loud stream of expletives, directed at Carol. Other people in the pool quickly moved to the side of the pool or got out, glancing at me with shocked, disbelieving expressions. Carol explained what had happened and why she was bringing me to the pool, but she had a hard time explaining while trying to watch me. It didn't happen frequently, but for some reason my head would fall down in the water, and I couldn't get it back up without Carol's help. Fortunately, after about three trips to the pool, Carol got me settled down so that I didn't curse. The water exercises were extremely helpful, and I gained strength in my arms and legs daily.

Kathy worked five days a week but came regularly on weekends and evenings to take care of Carol's children so that Carol had some time for herself or more time to spend with me. Everyone in the family worked well as a team.

Carol continued to take me for drives to the state park near her home. She packed a picnic lunch for us to sit in the car and share, but this was also a learning experience. Before I was allowed to eat, she said, "This is bread—say bread. This is lunchmeat—say lunchmeat. This is a cookie—say cookie," and so on. Wow! When I thought she was nearly finished with my lesson, I was like a corkscrew ready to pop. I stuffed that sandwich into my mouth with pure delight. Food wasn't my first priority anymore, but it was still mighty good.

I learned exceptionally fast. Even though I still showed child-like behavior, I didn't need to learn like a child, which is often through repetition. A psychologist who tried hypnosis to bring back my memory told me that everything I had learned in my lifetime was stored in my brain, and all I needed was a way to let it out. Hypnosis didn't work for me, but Carol found ways to bring out what I had learned. She also released an abundance of language skills and thinking processes.

For Family and Caregivers

Encourage your loved one to be as independent as possible.

- Allow him/her to make decisions as long as there's no safety risk.

- Find leisure activities for him/her

- Arrange for him/her to attend small, quiet, slow-paced social gatherings and fun activities.

- Play humorous movies, CDs and DVDs.

Be prepared for advances and setbacks

Expect slow progress. It took a year for me to be able to return to work and ten years before I felt completely recovered.

CHAPTER 9:

A Funny Story

*Everything is funny as long as it is happening
to someone else.*
Will Rogers

Perhaps this story was not funny to my family,
but later on, it was to me. When I first became
conscious, my mind seemed to be caught in a time
period many years earlier. When I saw a candy bar for
$.50, I was shocked; in my mind, it should have cost
$.05. When I saw pieces of candy at two for $.25, I
was extremely upset. They should cost $.01! Elated
with the success that Carol was having with me, my
father came up with a suggestion. He proposed that
he and mother take Carol and me to a restaurant for
lunch. Being a religious man and a frugal survivor of
the Great Depression, he was about to receive a shock.

He chose a modest restaurant, and I can still see his
broad smile as he helped me limp to a table. He gave
me the menu, because I was learning to read fairly
well, and asked me to choose what I'd like to eat. After

looking at the menu for a few minutes, my father and mother were horrified when I bellowed, "Let's get the h- out of here. It's too expensive!"

The waitress came running over to our table with an alarmed look on her face and said, "We have some very good specials today. They're written on that board over there."

My father quickly took my hand and in a soft voice said, "Judy, I knew how much things cost here before we came. I have enough money, so I want you to choose what you would like. Don't worry about the price." After that, I was quiet.

Carol had a hard time holding back a smile, because she had heard several of these expletives before!

Through humor, you can soften some of the worst blows that life delivers. And once you find laughter, no matter how painful your situation might be, you can survive it.
Bill Cosby

To Family and Caregivers

A brain injury is serious, but humor is always appropriate and helpful for the injured and caregiver. The positive image *you* portray can be the difference between healing and hindering recovery. Research and clinical trials have proven that humor is a powerful force that cannot be observed by the five senses, but its effects are consistent and undeniable. Don't force lengthy bouts of humor, but use it when your loved one is receptive. Use brief humor frequently.

- Keep some children's toys around for your loved one to play with.

- Create a humor file with funny cartoons, sayings and jokes to share with her/him.

- Take your loved-one (if able) to some old places she/he enjoyed as a child, like the zoo or an amusement park.

- Invite friends over for a "come-as-you-are" party or costume party.

- Invite children to visit.

- Interaction with dogs can be beneficial.

- Show humorous movies and listen to humorous CDs.

- Find leisure activities for her/him.

Humor resources include the following:

- American Association for Therapeutic Humor (AATH), California President: Steve Sultonoff

- Steve Wilson, Psychologist, Cheerman of the Bored of World Laughter Tours, Inc. and USA

Laughter Clubs, 1-800-669-5233 or www. stevewilson.com.

- Watch "Patch Adams," a movie starring Robin Williams, the true story of a physician who helped patients by making them laugh.

- Barnes & Noble Bookstores: Humor Section

CHAPTER 10:

Independence

*The greatest good you can do for another is not just to
share your riches but to reveal to him his own.*
Benjamin Disraeli

I stretched, rolled over in bed and loudly announced,
"I'm going home." No one heard me. I crawled out
of bed onto the floor and rigidly moved myself across
the floor by lying on my side, using my left hand and
foot to push my body along. I planned to get to the
living room to make my joyous announcement. No
one was there. I crawled on through the living room
and saw Carol in the kitchen.

My heart pounded with joy as I burst out with my
news, "I'm going home." Carol, in her usual pleasant
way, came over to me, smiled and helped me stand
up. Leaning against her with my right side, I limped
to a chair. By then, I was out of breath, but I couldn't
wait to emphatically repeat my announcement. Carol
hadn't reacted the first time. "I'm going home," I
burst out. Carol patted me on the arm and said, "I

have some good cereal this morning—just got a new one at the store." I shouted again, "I'm going home."

Carol sat down with me and gently said, "Judy, you can't go home yet. You can't cook. You can't dress yourself. You stay with me a little longer and soon you'll be ready, but not right now." I was furious and shouted again, "I'm going home!"

I must have been persistent or persuasive, because soon everyone was making plans for my return home. I lived on a main road in a rural area on four acres of land, somewhat secluded from other homes. Carol believed I needed a dog, not only for protection but for companionship, so off we went to the dog pound. We found the perfect dog. He was beautiful, part German Shepherd and part Labrador Retriever. While Carol and my father talked to him, he stood still with his tail between his legs, then walked away from them and gracefully sauntered over to me, nudged my hand with his nose, and started to wag his tail. I felt the connection immediately. I leaned down to pet him and he looked up, joyfully, into my eyes. From that moment on, we were friends. I named him Teddy, and away we went, Teddy and I sitting close in the back seat, with a broad smile on my face.

My beautiful daughter, Kimberly, came home from college to stay with me. She cooked, washed clothes, cleaned the house, and helped me get dressed, but Carol was still in charge. She encouraged Kimberly to read to me and talk to me about our shared experiences. Kimberly told me of vacations we had spent in

New Orleans, Disney World, and Ocean City. Carol came every day to continue my lessons, and then off we went to the pool. Soon the pool exercises allowed me to walk with a cane and the support of furniture, arranged strategically so that it allowed me to get to the bathroom and kitchen table. Carol arranged for a hospital bed to be placed in my living room, and Kimberly slept on the couch next to me. I had everything I needed, and I was gradually becoming independent.

Carol and others praised me, telling me that I was doing a wonderful job living by myself. Even though my brain was still clouded and my memory limited, I understood the importance of Kimberly and Carol in my life. Carol was the one who stimulated my brain, forced me in her kind way to do what I resisted, provided encouragement, and trained my body to function again. Without her, I would have lived like the doctors had surmised, as a "vegetable". Kimberly patiently helped me to care for myself and, most importantly, gave me her love.

Although my parents loved me as much as Carol, they expressed their love by doing *for* me, while Carol expressed her love by teaching me how to do for *myself*. She will always be my dearly beloved sister, my liberator, my miracle.

Our chief want in life is somebody who will make us do
what we can.
Ralph Waldo Emerson

Carol was that somebody!

CHAPTER 11:

Back to Work

*The ultimate measure of a man is not where he stands in a
moment of comfort and convenience, but where he stands at
times of challenge and controversy.*
Martin Luther King, Jr.

I was so proud. I was walking with a cane, dressing
myself and heating TV dinners in the microwave.
Kimberly had returned to school. My dog, Teddy, and
I were entertaining each other and feeling proud that
we were now completely independent.

My heart beat wildly when I was seated in my car
and fear engulfed me. My hands and arms were tense
and rigid as I carefully chose the position to place my
hands on the steering wheel. The sound of the motor
starting made my heart pound so fast and loud that I
could almost feel my chest shake. This fear never left
while I was driving, but the satisfaction of being able
to drive alone outweighed the constant fear.

My son, David, was satisfied that I was able to drive
alone. He had been coming home on weekends, taking

me to a large parking area in the local state park and going through the mechanics and skills of driving. I had mastered all the physical skills, but when he asked me where we were going, I never answered because I was not cognizant of the answer. "Are you turning right or left out of the driveway, Mom?" There was dead silence. "What road are we on?" Silence. "Where are we going, Mom?" Silence. Then, to his amazement, I made the correct turns, took the correct routes, and ended up at Bar Camp State Park where I apparently wanted to go.

As he became comfortable with my driving abilities, my decision making and knowledge of the road, he started allowing me to drive through small towns, then bigger towns, and finally to my place of employment. I was always able to go where David asked me to go or where I wanted to go, but I could never verbalize the route.

Carol had checked the federal law and found that disabled workers had to be given reasonable accommodations concerning reemployment, so she talked to my CEO to see if he would take me back in my old job, without pay, to see if I could do it. She found that he had temporarily filled my position with a close friend of mine, who was eager to have me fill the position again. She would back me up if I ran into problems.

My first day back was one of the most wonderful days of my life and at the same time one of the most frightening. I drove myself, came through the entrance alone, and walked up the steps to my office. The CEO and my friend were there waiting for me. They didn't know how to act and neither did I, but after a few moments, we greeted each other with open arms, and I cried with joy. My friend took me around to see all the people working that day. I recognized most of the faces but was unable to put names with them, so my friend had to help me recall the name of each person I encountered. She went over the daily duties with me as she did them and began to allow me to take her place. I learned quickly, and after several weeks, she put me back in charge.

Memory – memory – memory. I had little, so I carried around an 8" x 11" tablet and scribbled down almost everything anyone told me. I was sure I was fooling everyone. They thought I had a memory until one day a friend said, "Judy, you never used to forget anything, but now you don't remember anything." It wasn't said out of meanness or anger, rather sort of a joke, but I was flabbergasted and devastated. That did it! From then on, I took my notes home every night, reorganized them, and connected them. I don't know whether that helped or not, but it gave me more confidence, and no one ever teased me again.

Teddy was my confidant. I could tell him everything. If my day had been bad (like the day the person said I didn't remember anything), I told Teddy, and he understood. His tail went down, he looked into my eyes, lowered his head, and cuddled up close to me as I flopped down on my couch. When my day went great, I shared my joy with him. He jumped up and down like a little puppy and sometimes twirled around on a high jump. We were great buddies and friends.

Work went on this way, with its ups and downs. One day, the CEO called me into his office and told me that he was officially reinstating me into my position—with pay! I thought, "He must think I'm normal!" "Teddy, Teddy," I yelled when I got home, "let's celebrate!"

For Family and Caregivers

Federal law requires that disabled workers be given reasonable accommodations concerning reemployment.

- Meet with your doctor to determine what restrictions your loved one may have and what accommodations will be needed for him/her to return to work.

- Contact his/her previous place of employment and meet with the Human Resources director to discuss his/her return to work.

If you are unable to return to a previous job, go to the Internet and search for "job opportunities for head injured" or www.headinjury.com/jobs.htm.

Veterans: If you are unable to return to previous employment, consult the following:

- Go to the Internet and search for "job opportunities for veterans."

- Go to www.Military.com. It covers job search, a benefits guide, and VA Loans.

- Go to www.recruitmilitary.com for assistance.

- Go to usmilitary.about.com/od/job opportunities/military.

- Contact the Bob Woodruff Family Foundation at info@bobwoodrufffamilyfund.org.

- If dealing with Post-Traumatic Stress Disorder, call the National Center for Post Traumatic Stress Disorder (NCPTSD) at 802-296-6300.

- For veterans with disabilities needing rehabilitation, contact the National Rehabilitation Information Center (NRIC) at 800-346-2742 or www.naric.com.

Chapter 12:

Loneliness

*I don't think of all the misery but of the beauty
that still remains.*
Anne Frank

*L*oneliness, isolation, and depression often follow a severe brain injury. My old friends used to flock to my door, and everyone was happy to see me. They brought flowers and candy, and they kissed and patted me. After the brain injury, I smiled because I sensed that their presence was good. They smiled, and I smiled, but my mind was empty. Some of the faces were familiar, but I didn't know names. Gradually, they stopped coming.

I was truly feeling independent, but I was alone. I walked with only a slight limp and was still somewhat unsteady on my feet, sometimes appearing intoxicated because I staggered. People who knew me realized that I was not drunk, but they still seemed to keep their distance.

I walked around the mall several times a week "for exercise," but it was more to relieve my terrible loneliness. Weekends were exuberantly shared with family, but then I walked into my house alone— not just physically but mentally. Memories of my children's birthdays no longer existed. I don't know when they took their first steps, who their friends were, what they did in school, and how they looked going to the prom. I couldn't remember my first husband and our divorce—was it congenial or bitter? Although I laughed when my family told me funny stories about the past, I went home and wept, because I had no recollection of these prior happenings. I couldn't relate to the people I worked with, because I couldn't remember anything that we had shared.

Kimberly and David came home on as many weekends as they could. They took me to the places of my childhood wishes like the zoo, the ice cream store, a carnival, and shopping. Carol encouraged me to read books about other people with brain injuries, which she found through the BIAA bookstore as well as the pamphlet, "Helping Ourselves: Brain Injury Support Group."

A chance meeting ended my loneliness. One day on my lunch break, I went to the post office to buy stamps. There I saw a familiar face, but as usual, I didn't know his name. He spoke to me, smiled, and seeing my blank stare, introduced himself. He was Jim Powell, a classmate of mine from grades one through high school. I smiled, genuinely happy to see him.

One day, as I sat in my office, something prompted me to call him. A woman answered the phone—was it his wife? Horror struck! I explained that I was an old classmate of his who had had an accident resulting in a memory loss, and I wanted to meet with him to see if he could tell me things about school that might bring back some memories.

Much to my relief, the woman said, "I'm his mother. He's out of town right now, and I'm answering his business phone for him. May I tell him who called?" I said, "My name is Judy. Thank you."

I was horrified! What had I done? I had been taught that women never call men. I was so ashamed! I swore to myself that I'd never do anything like that again. Days went by, and my phone rang at work. It was Jim!

We went out for dinner, and I learned that he'd been divorced for eight years, the same as I had been. After dinner, he took me dancing, and we had lunch every day thereafter. We were married on November 23, 1984. My loneliness was gone, and I was starting a new life with new memories.

Jim was, and is, good for me. He is like Orpheus of Greek mythology, who was a poet, singer, and musician. His beautiful songs and inspiring music made trees uproot themselves, boulders melt, and rivers change their courses. His singing and music kept all those around him lighthearted and spirited. The story of his love for Eurydice shows that even when the most dark and painful experiences come into our lives, they can sometimes be a means to a better way forward.

My accident was the impetus leading to a new life and a better way forward. I've gained an enduring appreciation for natural beauty and the goodness of people, a special everlasting love for my sister Carol, my children, parents, family and, now, my wonderful husband, Jim.

For Family and Caregivers

- Start a brain injury support group for your loved one to help relieve his/ her loneliness.

- Order "Helping Ourselves: Brain Injury Support Group" from the BIAA at www.biausa.org.

- On the Internet, search for "brain injury support group."

- Consider participating in a research project and contact the BIAA at www.biausa.org.

- For injured soldiers:

- Contact your nearest VA hospital and inquire about soldier support groups.

- Go to www.Military.com and click on "Buddy Finder."

CHAPTER 13:
My Secret Miracle

If I lived a billion years more, in my body or yours, there's
not a single experience on Earth that could ever be
as good as being dead. Nothing.
Dr. Dianne Morrissey

*I*didn't tell anyone about this "miracle" because I
was afraid anyone who heard it would think I was
crazy. After nearly a year, however, I found the courage to tell Carol. She listened attentively and gently
assured me that I was not crazy.

I said, "I was caught up in a bright, peaceful
place that was moving me along toward something I
couldn't see. I had a calm, happy feeling. As I moved
along, I could see nothing except brightness, but I
knew it was very beautiful. Then I was surrounded by
many faceless, bodiless, kind, good forms that were
like people, but were not people, welcoming me. They
made me feel wanted and loved. It was the most wonderful experience I'd ever known. I try to describe it as
beautiful, wonderful, glorious, but there are truly no

words to describe it. Gradually it ended and I cried. I wanted to stay there."

Carol told me that she had been with me the day before I awoke. She said that I moaned and for the first time cried out, "Let me go." My voice was weak and tears poured from my eyes as I repeated, "Let me go" several times before reverting back into a coma.

"It is truly a miracle, Judy. You may have had an out-of-body or near-death-experience, which has been written about by many." She smiled and said, "You may have gone to heaven."

It was a strong experience, one that has given me a rich, secure feeling about death. Death, as I believe I experienced it, is a beautiful part of life. It is something to look forward to rather than fear. It is a calm, natural part of living.

CHAPTER 14:

New Memories

Nobody can go back and start a new beginning, but anyone
can start today and make a new ending.
Maria Robinson

After losing nearly forty-two years of a happy child-hood, marriage, children, and work memories, I am living a new life with extraordinary new memories of love and happiness. They can never replace my early memories, but they certainly enrich my life now.

One of my most precious memories is the gift Jim gave me for my retirement. He took me, our five children, their spouses, and our eleven grandchildren to Hawaii for the most wonderful trip I've ever had.

Jim and I wanted to make happy memories for ourselves and grandchildren, so we started annual New Year's Eve and St. Patrick's Day parties. The parties always had the same agenda. We shared a child-friendly dinner and then started a plethora of activities. The children were given a blank, white t-shirt to decorate with magic markers, and then they made paper hats and decorated them with feathers, beads, and stickers. After the quiet time of working on their creations, we enthusiastically marched around the house to Sousa marches—the changing leader wielded a baton and made gyrations mimicked by the followers, which included me and Jim. After marching, we rolled, cut, and decorated sugar cookies. While I was baking them, Jim played games and awarded a prize to each child. We then danced the Macarena, the Chicken Dance, and the Hokey Pokey. It was then time for the grand finale!

We all donned our newly created shirts and hats, chose our noise makers, and formed a circle. While Jim counted to ten, little eyes gleamed, and mouths curled in big grins. At the count of ten, we all shouted, as loud as we could, "Happy New Year" or "Happy St. Patrick's Day," blew the horns, and rattled our noise makers. We all kissed each other and ran to the kitchen for cookies and milk. After much talking about the fun they'd had, with fingers and mouths wiped clean, their little eyes began to droop, and each child was lovingly tucked in bed.

The next morning after breakfast, they were allowed to watch children's videos while Jim and I prepared lunch for them and their returning parents. What great fun it was for me, hearing them eagerly tell their moms and dads about their activities. What happy memories I had years later when our grandchildren reminisced about these parties.

We also formed memories by taking each grandchild to a restaurant of his/her choice for his birthday, watching him/her open a gift, and sharing an evening of entertainment. As the children grew older and we were no longer "hip" enough to choose appropriate gifts, their entertainment was shopping with us for their own birthday gifts. We were pleased when one of our college-age grandchildren, on his birthday, requested a return trip to the same restaurant where he'd spent his childhood birthdays.

Many other wonderful memories have filled my life over twenty-three years. Jim and I traveled to Hawaii, England, France, Holland, East and West Germany, Yugoslavia, Hungary, Italy, Switzerland, China, and Russia. These trips provided marvelous memories of sites, information, and the goodness and individualism of people all around the world.

I changed employment to be nearer our adult children, who were marrying and starting families. Jim was in business for himself, so he was able to continue his business and start a branch in our new location.

I took a position as director of ambulatory care for a hospital in mid-Ohio and was promoted to vice president of patient care services. I worked in this hospital for fifteen years until I retired, and have many precious memories of those "normal" years.

CHAPTER 15:
Normal Pressure Hydrocephalus (NPH)

Sometimes in our confusion, we see not the world as it is, but
the world through eyes blurred by the mind.
Anonymous

It was 2004, twenty-three years after my brain injury and a few days before my retirement. I was experiencing some strange occurrences. I had guests coming for dinner, and one hour before they arrived, as I began to set the dinner table, I panicked because I thought I had no dishes. I raced to the attic, unpacked some old china, hurriedly washed it, and set the table. The rest of the evening went as usual with the guests, but the next morning, I saw my china in the china closet and began to laugh. How could I have forgotten about my good china? I told Jim how silly I'd been, and we laughed. I told him about forgetting my daughter's phone number, and we laughed again.

Fortunately for us, I had my yearly physical exam about a week later. After concluding that everything looked all right on the exam, my physician asked if anything new had been happening. Addressing him as the friend he'd become, I laughingly told him about forgetting my dishes, and his smile faded. He said, "I'd like to send you to a neurologist. I don't think there is anything wrong, but I just want to make sure."

I got to see the neurologist quickly, and he asked me, "Do you have trouble holding your urine?"

"Yes, but my mother has had the same problem, so I think it is hereditary."

"Are you having difficulty walking?"

"I don't think so."

Jim jumped in and told the doctor, "She has been walking slowly, like she can't lift her feet off the ground. Our daughter and I took her to the fair, and we had to keep stopping and waiting for her to catch up with us. She's usually leading us around." The neurologist ordered a CT scan, an MRI, and cisternogram, (a nuclear test used to diagnose spinal fluid circulation problems).

When he received the results, much to my surprise and confusion, the neurologist told me that I had NPH. "NPH is excess fluid in the brain, which causes people to have difficulty lifting their feet to walk, makes them unable to hold their urine, and causes severe memory loss. It can occur fairly quickly or gradually over time. Often people who have had a brain injury, like you, develop NPH. Sometimes it is not correctly diagnosed, and doctors think it's Alzheimer's or Parkinson's, because the symptoms can be very similar. If left untreated, it can be completely debilitating, but fortunately there is a treatment that has been successful. A neurosurgeon can go into a ventricle of your brain and place a shunt, which is connected to a tube threaded down through your neck and chest into your abdomen. This shunt drains the excess fluid from your brain into your abdomen where it is eliminated by natural means. As soon as the fluid is eliminated, people return almost immediately to their normal self. I've already scheduled you with a neurosurgeon."

I thought back to a couple of months at work before I retired. I had turned over most of my responsibilities to my replacement, so I thought that my short-term memory loss was happening because I didn't have that much to remember anymore. I also noticed that I had trouble walking quickly but thought it must be psychological, because maybe I didn't want to retire— though I knew I did!

Soon, I couldn't remember my wonderful retirement trip to Hawaii. Why couldn't I remember any of it? I became completely incoherent. I thought Jim was my first husband and his sisters were my ex sister-in-laws. I repeated nonsensical questions over and over: "Are we going to Grandma's house?" As I became more disoriented, Jim contacted the neurosurgeon to see when my surgery was scheduled and found that it was planned for several months later. When Jim explained my condition, the surgeon moved the date up. I soon underwent the surgery, and much to my and Jim's delight, I returned to normal.

I sent this letter to my friends after the surgery:

Dear Friends,

This is to thank you and let you know how much I appreciated your cards and good wishes. I also want to write to share information with you about my condition and surgery, so that you may help someone you know or love who may have a similar condition.

My condition was called Normal Pressure Hydro-cephalus (NPH). It is caused by excess fluid build-ing up in the ventricles of the brain. It may progress slowly over a period of months or years, but then the crippling symptoms finally occur. Some literature says they think it's common in people who've had a stroke or brain injury, but it also occurs in others. The symptoms include difficulty walking and lifting the legs, which may be thought to be arthritis or Par-kinson's disease. Memory loss progresses to a point of not knowing who your relatives are or where you live. You are oriented to the times you lived many years before. Asking the same questions repeatedly without grasping the answer is common. All these symptoms may be attributed to Alzheimer's disease or some other mental state. A loss of bladder control is common. If you know of someone with these symptoms, he/she needs to see a neurologist and have a CT scan, MRI, and a cisternogram. These tests make the correct diagnosis clear. Once the diagnosis is made, a neurosurgeon will place a shunt in a ventricle of the brain connected to a tube, which is threaded down through the neck and chest into the abdomen. The excess fluid is eliminated, and the symptoms begin to disappear immediately.

I feel blessed that I saw a neurologist who checked me for this problem. I was referred to him because I had a period of memory loss (couldn't remember where my dishes in the kitchen were when I was having guests for dinner, so I went to the attic and unpacked some old dishes that I had stored there). The next day, I was fine and laughed at myself for being so silly. Fortunately, I saw my family doctor shortly after that for a routine checkup. When I told him the embarrassing story, he referred me to a neurologist right away. I had also had difficulty walking for some time, which my doctor and I thought was arthritis. Urine leaks forced me to wear pantyliners, but other female friends of mine said that this is common in women of my age, and it was also true of my mother, so I thought little of it. Before my surgery could be scheduled, I had developed all the other symptoms related to not knowing who, what, or where I was.

I understand that this is a relatively new diagnosis and many doctors don't know about it, so the patient's family or friends may have to help the person find a knowledgeable neurologist. You can find a specialist in your area who can diagnose and treat NPH by going to www.lifenph.com. Click on "Five Steps to Diagnosis and Treatment" and then on "physician location."

You may have seen an ad on TV with an elderly man who explains the symptoms and the name of the condition. I've been told that this man was completely incapacitated and needed constant care for several years before his condition was correctly diagnosed. Like me, he wants to tell the world about it, because it is so relatively easy to cure.

Please share what I've told you with all your friends and relatives with the hope that you may save others from a misdiagnosis of Alzheimer's or Parkinson's or living a handicapped life and being a burden to their families. Thank you once again for your kindness.

Love, Judy

Only one thing disappeared with my NPH and didn't come back: my self-confidence. I wanted to write a book about my sister's success in rehabilitating me after my brain injury, but I had lost the confidence to do it.

For Family and Caregivers

For more information on NPH:

- Hydrocephalus Association
  4340 East West Highway, Suite 905
  Bethesda, MD 20814
  Phone: 301-202-3811
          888-598-3789
  Fax: 301-202-3813
  www.hydroassoc.org and info@hydroassoc.org

- For Neurosurgeons and Neurologists who treat
  adult hydrocephalus and NPH, go to
  Hydrocephalus Association:
  click Normal Pressure
  Hydrocephalus, scroll down to
  HA's Online NPH Resources,
  see Online Directory of
  Neurosurgeons and
  Neurologists Who Treat Adults

- Codman: www.lifenph.com

The Hydrocephalus Association estimates that
375,000 older Americans suffer from NPH. This figure
may be low because of the number of misdiagnoses.
It is often confused with Alzheimer's and Parkinson's
disease.

CHAPTER 16:

Restoration of Confidence

If you hear a voice within you saying, "You are not a painter," then by all means paint and that voice will be silenced.
Vincent Van Gogh

*I*t had been three years since my recovery from NPH, but I still felt inadequate. I wanted to write, but each time I thought of it, I felt depressed. What would I say? How would I begin? What would I include? The unanswered questions plagued me.

Jim woke up one morning on a snowy, cold Ohio day, looked out the window, and said, "Let's go to Florida and get out of this weather." I laughed, but he said, "I mean it. Let's go!"

He unlocked his "touring brain" and started researching and planning. I call it his "touring brain" because he's taken me on so many outstanding trips. He came up with plans to sightsee and visit four friends in Florida, one of them being Julie Moore, who had read to me while I was in a coma. Off we went! One stop was to visit our daughter-in-law's parents, who lived in an over 55 community called Betmar in Zephyrhills. We found we loved it there, and they introduced us to many of their friends and activities.

The next year, during the cold Ohio winter, we made the same trip to Florida. That time we were able to rent a place in Betmar for two weeks. I found a writers' group there and went to one of its meetings. The people were as nice as they could be, but they overwhelmed me with the quality of their writing. They had each written a short essay and took turns reading them. When it came to me, of course, I was unprepared and had to admit that I had nothing to read. Everyone joined in making me feel welcome and voiced their understanding, as this was my first meeting. Their writing seemed so good that I felt even more inadequate.

I looked forward to returning to beautiful, sunny Florida the next year. We had arranged to rent a place in Betmar for three months, and during the first month, January, I felt uncomfortable and sad. I missed our children and others. I wasn't excited about joining any of the activities, but my wonderful Jim said, "I want you to write a short part of your book and take it to the writers group." He had to say no more. I stopped feeling sorry for myself. I wrote and went to the next Creative Writers Club of Betmar meeting.

I was greeted with a smile from every member as they welcomed me and introduced themselves. After I read my piece, they applauded when I finished and made complimentary comments about phrases I'd used. I was elated! I continued to write and to receive kind, constant encouragement. They restored my self-confidence and gave me the courage to keep writing. I wrote a poem to thank them for all they did for me and have included it in this book.

CHAPTER 17:

Goodness That Emerged from Bad

*God's way of answering the Christians' prayer for
more patience, experience, hope, and love often is to put
him in the furnace of affliction.
Richard Cecil*

My head injury, handicaps, and NPH may be considered bad experiences, but much more good than bad has come from them. Let me share some of the good with you.

The Beauty of Nature

Waking up from a coma allowed me to see the world for the first time, not as a child who gradually becomes aware of his/her surroundings but as an adult who sees all the wonder in one moment. When I was taken outdoors, the world looked breathtakingly beautiful. I felt small, like a tiny flower petal being bathed in warm, silky, soft wisps of air, and the world around me was majestic. I marveled at the beautiful, blue sky with filmy, white clouds billowing in many shades of gray and white. I saw a tree, standing tall and straight, its delicate leaves of shaded green shimmering in the wind. I felt the soft, velvet touch of a rose petal, smelled the sweet aroma of orange blossoms, and saw a butterfly emerging from a larva. Seeing the world around me for the first time filled me with awe and eternal appreciation.

The Love of People

I was filled with happiness each time I saw people's lips curl into a smile. Whether they came from someone known or unknown, each was beautiful to me. Smiles gave me a sense of well being, pleasure and being loved. Academic literature indicates that brain-injured people respond more successfully to a loved one rather than an unknown professional, and I believe this was true for me. At home, I was surrounded by the love of my sisters, father and mother, my children, family and friends, and my dear new husband. Their love motivated me, and I wanted to please them and respond to their instructions and urgings. Total strangers from the Betmar Creative Writers Club, with love and acceptance, restored my confidence in myself and my writing. I am convinced that love healed me.

*The cure for all ills and wrongs, the cares, the sorrows,
and the crimes of humanity, all lie in one word "love".
It is the divine vitality that everywhere produces and
restores life. To each and every one of us, it gives the
power of working miracles if we will.*
Lydia Maria Child

The Power of Prayer

Carol prayed for wisdom and found ways to make me well. God answered. Prayer provided me with comfort and the friendship of God when I experienced loneliness. I've learned that nothing is as powerful as prayer.

*Ask, and it shall be given to you; seek and ye shall find;
knock and it shall be opened unto you.*
Matthew 7:7

Family and Friends

Brain injuries take longer to heal than the rehabilitation time provided by insurance. I've experienced invaluable assistance from family and friends, and I am living proof that their efforts and love resulted in my recovery. They pushed, encouraged, motivated, insisted, and assisted me to do what rehabilitation professionals recommended. I had no understanding of or motivation to do what needed to be done, but *they* did.

My Lesson Learned

I've learned that our world is made up of good and bad. They both happen to all of us, but we see them differently. If we look for the good, we find it and if we look for the bad, we also find it. My "bad" experience opened my eyes to an unbelievable amount of good. I encourage you to look for the good!

Addendum A

Organizations to assist the underprivileged and foreign speakers.

For the Indigent

Rancho Los Amigos National Rehabilitation Center
7601 East Imperial Highway, Downy, CA 90242
www.rancho.org

For Foreign Speakers

Promotes communication among family and head-injured persons in ten different languages.

The Perspectives Network, Inc.
P.O. Box 121012,
W. Melbourne, FL 32912-1012
www.tbi.org

Addendum B

Organizations with head/brain injury information and assistance. Brain/head injuries and strokes are similar, and the information about strokes may be helpful.

Brain Injury Association
 of America (BIAA)
1608 Spring Hill Road,
Suite 110
Vienna, VA 22182
703-761-0750

www.biausa.org
State affiliates
(see Addendum D)
1-800-444-6443
for Brain Injury Infor-
mation only

Brain Injury Resource
 Center
PO Box 84151
Seattle, WA 98124-5451
Head Injury Hotline:

Brain@headinjury.com
www.headinjury.com

206-621-8558

National Rehabilitation
 Information Center
8201 Corporate Drive,
 Suite 600
Landover, MD 20785

1-800-346-2742

www.naric.com

National Stroke Association
9707 E. Easter Lane
Centennial, CO 80112

1-800-787-6537

National Family
   Caregivers Association
10400 Connecticut Ave.
Kensington, MD
   20895-3944

www.nfcacares.org

1-800-896-3650

Defense and Veterans
   Brain Injury Center
   (DVBIC)
National Headquarters
1335 East-West Highway,
   Ste. 6-100
Silver Spring, MD 20910

www.DVBIC.org

1-800-870-9244

Outreach Call Center:
   1-866-966-1020

Rainbow Rehabilitation
   Centers
38777 Six Mile Road
   Suite 101
Livonia, MI 48152

1-800-968-6644

Rainbow Visions
   Magazine
Head Injury Hotline

www.rainbowvisions-
magazine.com
206-621-8558

Addendum C

See information available from:

Brain Injury Association of America (BIAA) at www.biausa.org.

Go to above website. Click on "Marketplace" at top of screen, then click "Booklets" at the left.

"Facts about the Vegetative and Minimally Conscious States After Brain Injury"

"Living with Brain Injury Booklets" (the five listed below may be purchased in a set or individually)

1. "Behavioral Challenges after Brain Injury"

2. "Challenges, Changes, and Choices: A Brain Injury Guide for Families and Caregivers"

3. "A Physician Speaks about Severe Brain Injury"

4. "Falls and Traumatic Brain Injury: The Basics"

5. "Driving after Brain Injury: Issues, Obstacles, and Possibilities

"Living with Brain Injury Booklet 2005"

Employment, Depression, and Substance Abuse

"Living With Brain Injury Booklet 2006, Overcoming Loneliness, Building Lasting Relationships"

"Communicating with an Adult after Brain Injury"

"Living with Brain Injury: A Guide for Families with a Child with a Brain Injury"

The Essential Brain Injury Guide

Addendum D

Brain Injury Association of America
Chartered State Affiliates

Brain Injury Association of Arizona	602-323-9165 - 888-500-9165
Brain Injury Association of Arkansas	501-374-3585 - 800-235-2443
Brain Injury Association of California	661-872-4903
Brain Injury Association of Colorado	303-355-9969 - 800-955-2443
Brain Injury Association of Connecticut	860-721-8111 - 800-278-8242
Brain Injury Association of Delaware	800-411-0505
Brain Injury Association of Florida	850-410-0103 - 800-992-3442
Brain Injury Association of Georgia	404-712-5504

Brain Injury Association of Hawaii	808-454-0699
Brain Injury Association of Idaho	208-342-0999 - 888-374-3447
Brain Injury Association of Illinois	312-726-5699 - 800-699-6443
Brain Injury Association of Indiana	317-356-7722 - 866-854-4246
Brain Injury Association of Iowa	511-244-5606 - 800-444-6443
Brain Injury Association of Kansas	816-842-8607 - 800-783-1356
Brain Injury Association of Kentucky	502-493-0609 - 800-592-1117
Brain Injury Association of Maine	207-861-9900 - 800-275-1233
Brain Injury Association of Maryland	410-448-2924 - 800-221-6443
Brain Injury Association of Massachusetts	508-475-0032 - 800-242-0030

Brain Injury Association
of Michigan

810-229-5880 -
800-772-4323

Brain Injury Association
of Minnesota

612-378-2742 -
800-669-6442

Brain Injury Association
of Mississippi

601-981-1021 -
800-641-6442

Brain Injury Association
of Missouri

314-426-4024 -
800-377-6442

Brain Injury Association
of Montana

406-541-6442 -
800-241-6442

Brain Injury Association
of New Hampshire

603-225-8400 -
800-773-8400

Brain Injury Association
of New Jersey

732-738-1002 -
800-669-4323

Brain Injury Association
of New Mexico

505-292-7414 -
888-292-7415

Brain Injury Association
of New York

518-459-7911 -
800-228-8201

Brain Injury Association
of North Carolina

919-833-9634 -
800-377-1464

Brain Injury Association of Ohio	614-481-7100 - 866-644-6242
Brain Injury Association of Oklahoma	580-233-4363
Brain Injury Association of Oregon	503-413-7707 - 800-544-5243
Brain Injury Association of Pennsylvania	717-657-3601 - 866-635-7097
Brain Injury Association of Rhode Island	401-461-6599
Brain Injury Association of South Carolina	803-731-9823 - 800-290-6461
Brain Injury Association of Tennessee	615-248-5878 - 877-757-2428
Brain Injury Association of Texas	512-326-1212 - 800-392-0040
Brain Injury Association of Utah	801-484-2240 - 800-281-8442
Brain Injury Association of Vermont	802-985-8440 - 877-856-1772

Brain Injury Association of Virginia	804-355-5748 - 800-334-8443
Brain Injury Association of Washington	253-238-6085 - 800-523-5438
Brain Injury Association of West Virginia	304-766-4892 - 800-356-6443
Brain Injury Association of Wisconsin	262-790-9660 - 800-882-9282
Brain Injury Association of Wyoming	304-473-1767 - 800-643-6457

Addendum E

Members of the Creative Writers Club of Betmar

Gail Tracy, President

Joyce Miller, Facilitator

Ed Russell, Secretary/Treasurer

Verna Thornton (my editor)

Carolyn Amos	Carl Kass
Mary Deland	Gordon Lord
Eglantine Ford	Tom Merchant
Freda Gladle	Louis Miller
Glen Goddard	Richard Phelan
Marilyn Reiff	Julius Greff
Mary Haggins	David Richardson
Betsy Hayba	Catherine Tirpko

Janet Verville

Addendum F

Poem for the Creative Writers Club Members

A mind lost
In shadows of
Uncertainty and doubt
A yearning for confidence and assurance

Then light from friendly faces
A handshake, a smile,
Compliments, support,
Renewed courage and confidence.

The bright sunshine of
A life restored with self-confidence.
Creativity, spirit, and faith.
A thank you to the writers of Betmar.

www.ingramcontent.com/pod-product-compliance
Lightning Source LLC
Chambersburg PA
CBHW060512280326
41933CB00014B/2938

GARLAND GENEALOGY

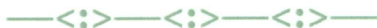

—<:>——<:>——<:>—

The Descendants

[The Northern Branch]

—of—

Peter Garland

Mariner

Admitted Resident of
Charlestown, Massachusetts Bay
in 1637

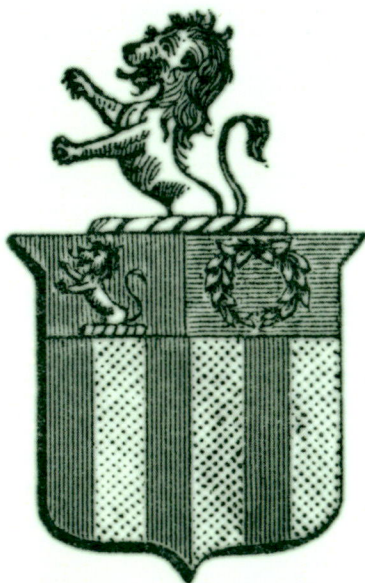

By *James Gray Garland*